Skin Tag Removal

Discover the Key to Achieving Radiant, Youthful Skin the Natural Way

Marvin Bernstein

Introducing the exclusive and captivating world of Marvin Bernstein. Immerse yourself in the timeless elegance and creativity that defines our brand. Experience the unparalleled craftsmanship and attention to detail that sets us apart. Discover the essence of sophistication and style with our exquisite collection.

Table of Contents

Preface

Do you find yourself frustrated by the sudden appearance of those bothersome skin tags? Are you seeking a solution for achieving clear, healthy skin, but find yourself inundated with a multitude of treatments and remedies? Get ready to experience a remarkable transformation as you dive into our innovative books that are set to completely revolutionize your skincare regimen.

Discover the Incredible Potential of Natural Healing

In a world filled with an overwhelming number of products and procedures that rely on chemicals and invasive methods, our books provide a refreshing alternative: the incredible potential of natural healing. We are firm believers in the power of nature to unlock the secrets to clear, radiant skin. With a blend of timeless wisdom and cutting-edge methods, we are here to lead you on a comprehensive path towards achieving vibrant and healthy skin.

Explore the Depths of Holistic Skincare Principles

Our books go beyond simply addressing skin tags; they focus on revolutionizing your skincare regimen holistically. Explore the depths of holistic skincare principles that tackle the underlying causes of skin problems, giving you the knowledge to make educated choices about your health and well-being. Our comprehensive guides offer valuable insights and practical tips to help you achieve lasting results, whether it's understanding the mind-body connection or adopting mindful skincare practices.

Uncover the Soothing Effects of Herbs and Essential Oils

Picture bidding farewell to costly creams and treatments and embracing the therapeutic potential of herbs and essential oils. Our books reveal the wonders of nature's pharmacy, providing do-it-yourself formulas and gentle remedies for removing skin tags. These solutions are not only safe and effective, but also kind to your skin. Discover the power of natural remedies for achieving healthy and glowing skin. Explore a variety of plant-based therapies, including lavender, tea tree oil, aloe vera, and witch hazel, and unlock their potential for a radiant complexion.

Purify and Revitalize Your Skin from the Inside Out

Our books provide valuable insights on achieving clear, radiant skin by focusing on natural cleansing and detoxification methods. Discover various detox diets, cleansing rituals, and supplements that can assist your body in naturally eliminating toxins and impurities, which may be linked to skin problems. By nourishing your body internally, you can effectively eliminate skin tags and reveal a radiant glow that emanates from within.

Nurture a Mindful Skincare Routine

Taking care of your skin goes beyond just applying products; it involves nurturing your body and mind as well. Our books highlight the significance of developing a mindful skincare routine that integrates stress reduction techniques, meditation, and self-care practices. By taking care of your inner well-being, you'll achieve a harmonious balance that will be reflected in your outward appearance. This will result in clear, radiant skin that showcases your confidence and vitality.

Revolutionary Solutions for Radiant, Youthful Skin

Are you prepared to start a transformative journey towards achieving radiant and rejuvenated skin? Our books offer reliable methods for removing skin tags that are both safe and scientifically proven to be effective. With our comprehensive resources, we provide you with detailed instructions, tips for aftercare, and strategies to prevent any issues along your skincare journey. Our goal is to help you achieve the desired results while prioritizing the health of your skin.

Authentic Narratives, Genuine Metamorphoses

However, it's important to note that we're not the only ones saying this. Our books are brimming with captivating tales of individuals who have completely revitalized their skin and lives by embracing the power of natural skincare methods. From conquering skin insecurities to embracing their innate beauty, their personal journeys demonstrate the transformative effects of a comprehensive skincare routine. By tapping into the knowledge and guidance of top skincare professionals, you'll be equipped with all the necessary tools to begin your personal quest for vibrant, blemish-free skin.

Begin your journey to glowing skin today

Are you prepared to tap into the full potential of your skin and uncover the hidden secrets to achieving naturally clear and radiant skin? It's time to bid farewell to skin tags and welcome a new era of skincare that embraces the beauty of nature. Our transformative books will take you on a journey to achieve clear, youthful skin that exudes health and vitality. Why wait any longer? Start your journey towards glowing skin today!

Introduction

Do you have enough of self-consciousness over those unsightly skin tags? "Skin Tag Removal: Your Comprehensive Guide to Clear, Radiant Skin" can help you choose the best treatment possible. Bid farewell to the aggravation and shame resulting from unattractive skin tags and welcome to a radiant, self-assured complexion.

Renowned skincare specialist Marvin Bernstein shares the keys to a secure and efficient skin tag removal procedure in this game-changing manual. With years of experience and knowledge under his belt, [Marvin Bernstein] offers comprehensive solutions and easy-to-follow guidelines to help you naturally attain clear, glowing skin.

This book has all the information you need to restore the health and vibrancy of your skin, from comprehending the underlying causes of skin tags to using tried-and-true removal methods. Learn how to permanently remove skin tags without the need for costly treatments or intrusive procedures by utilizing the power of natural substances and essential oils.

However, this book is about empowerment rather than merely removal. You are empowered by Marvin Bernstein to take charge of your skincare regimen and adopt a wholistic perspective on beauty. You may not only get rid of skin tags that are already there but also stop new ones from growing by following some useful advice on prevention and upkeep.

Enormous with enlightening counsel, motivational success stories, and doable tactics, "Skin Tag Removal" is your go-to manual for getting the clear, glowing skin of your dreams. This book is your guide to successful skincare, whether you're battling a few unsightly skin tags or a more serious problem.

Skin tags should no longer be a barrier to you. "Skin Tag Removal: Your Comprehensive Guide to Clear, Radiant Skin" is the first step towards a better, more assured future. Get it now. Your confidence and skin will both appreciate it.

Chapter 1

Discover the Secrets of Pores and Skin Tags!

Introducing the incredible epidermis/skin tags! These remarkable flesh-colored growths gracefully emerge around the surface of your skin. Suspended from a delicate stalk made of tissues, they are truly a sight to behold. Discover the fascinating world of human skin with its unique characteristics. Did you know that these growths, known as epidermis/skin tags, are actually quite common? In fact, a remarkable 25% of trusted resources reveal that many individuals have at least one of these intriguing skin tags. Embrace the diversity of your own skin!

Discover the secret of finding epidermis tags nestled within the folds of your skin in these specific areas:

- Introducing the revolutionary solution for underarm freshness - Armpits! Say goodbye to unwanted odors and hello to confidence with

Armpits, the ultimate underarm

- Introducing our revolutionary product that will change the way you experience comfort: the ComfortMax Body Wrap! Designed with your ultimate comfort in mind, our body wrap provides unparalleled support and relief in three key areas: the neck, under the breasts, and around the genitals. Say goodbye to discomfort and hello to pure bliss with the Comfort Body Wrap!

- Introducing a rare occurrence - the emergence of epidermis tags within the delicate confines of your eyelids.

- Introducing the remarkable Epidermis Tags! These little wonders may not cause any medical issues, but they can be quite bothersome when they rub against your clothes. Say goodbye to discomfort and hello to a world of relief with Epidermis Tags!

Experience the ultimate solution for removing skin tags on your eyelids.

Discover the freedom of choice when it comes to skin tags. No need to eliminate them unless they truly bother you. Embrace a life free from unnecessary concerns. Discover the multitude of options available to effortlessly eliminate those pesky epidermis tags, all in the name of enhancing your aesthetic appeal.

Introducing Home Treatments: The Ultimate Solution for Your Health and Wellness Needs

Discover the secret to effortlessly banishing unsightly epidermis/skin tags with the power of apple cider vinegar, as recommended by top websites. Discover the safe and effective way to remove skin tags with apple cider vinegar! But remember, it's always wise to consult with your trusted health-care professional before taking matters into your own hands. Protect your precious eye area from harm.

Discover the secret to effortlessly removing skin tags with ease. With our innovative method, you can gently tie off the base of your skin tag using dental floss or cotton, effectively cutting off its blood flow. Say goodbye to unsightly skin tags and hello to flawless skin! Experience the natural process of your skin layer tag gracefully shedding away. Discover the power of seeking advice from a trusted physician once more before embarking on this revolutionary system. Discover the secret to safely and effectively removing epidermis tags with our exceptional base solution. Say goodbye to the risks of excessive bleeding or infection. Discover the potential for leaving behind a flawless impression on your eyelid with our revolutionary product.

Discover the World of Cutting-Edge Medical Procedures and Transformative Treatments

Discover the safest way to remove those pesky epidermis tags by entrusting the task to a skilled health-care professional. With their expertise, they will employ the most effective techniques to eliminate those unwanted bits of skin from your delicate eyelid. Rest assured, this treatment will successfully address the existing skin tags you have. However, it's important to note that it won't provide a foolproof solution to prevent new epidermis tags from appearing in the future.

Experience the ultimate in rejuvenation with Cryotherapy.

Experience the power of cryotherapy, the cutting-edge treatment that harnesses the extreme chill to effortlessly freeze off unsightly epidermis/skin tags. With the skilled touch of a medical doctor, water nitrogen is delicately applied to your skin layer using a cotton swab or a precise pair of tweezers. Say goodbye to those bothersome skin tags and embrace a smoother, more flawless complexion. Experience the power of our revolutionary liquid solution as it delicately interacts with your skin. Feel a slight tingling sensation, a sign that our formula is actively working to address your skin concerns. Watch as your frozen pores and skin tags effortlessly dissolve, revealing a smoother, more radiant complexion. Within just ten days, you'll witness the remarkable transformation. Trust our innovative solution to deliver exceptional results.

Experience the transformative power of our drinking water nitrogen application. Witness the remarkable formation of a blister in your community, a testament to the effectiveness of our product. Rest assured, this blister will scab over and gracefully fall off within a fortnight to a month, leaving behind a revitalized and rejuvenated environment.

Experience the transformative power of surgical removal.

Discover a simple and effective method to eliminate those pesky skin tags - by delicately trimming them away. Experience the expertise of a skilled medical professional as they delicately numb the targeted area and effortlessly eliminate your skin tag using a precise scalpel or specialized medical scissors.

Experience the cutting-edge technology of Electrosurgery.

Experience the revolutionary power of electrosurgery, a cutting-edge technique that harnesses the gentle warmth to delicately melt away unsightly skin tags from the comfort of your own home. Say goodbye to those bothersome blemishes and hello to smooth, flawless skin. Try electrosurgery today and discover the transformative results for yourself. Introducing our revolutionary burning method - the ultimate solution to prevent excessive loss of blood when removing tags. Say goodbye to those painful moments and hello to a safer and more efficient experience. Trust our cutting-edge technology to keep you protected. Try it today!

Experience the Power of Ligation Discover the incredible process of ligation, where skilled physicians expertly tie off the base of your skin tag, effectively cutting off its blood flow. Experience the remarkable transformation of your skin tag as it gracefully withers away and effortlessly detaches itself from your skin in just a matter of weeks.

Discover the Fascinating Causes Behind Epidermis/Skin Tags on Eyelids!

Introducing skin tags, the result of a fascinating combination of collagen protein and arteries, delicately enveloped by a layer of epidermis. While the exact cause of these intriguing skin formations remains a mystery to the medical community, they tend to manifest in areas where the skin folds, such as the armpits, groin, or eyelids. It is believed that the friction caused by the gentle rubbing of skin against skin may play a role in their development.

Discover the unfortunate truth: individuals who struggle with excess weight are more likely to develop unsightly skin tags due to the presence of extra skin folds. Experience the transformative power of pregnancy as hormonal changes work their magic, potentially increasing the likelihood of those pesky epidermis/skin tags making an appearance. And that's not all - there could even be a fascinating connection between insulin resistance, diabetes, and the formation of these intriguing epidermis tags. Prepare to be amazed!

Discover the natural phenomenon that occurs as people gracefully age - an increase in epidermis/skin tags. These unique growths tend to make their appearance during the middle generation and beyond, adding character and charm to the skin. Discover the fascinating world of epidermis/skin tags, where genetics play a captivating role. Uncover the intriguing possibility that these delightful epidermis growths may be passed down through generations, bestowing upon certain individuals an elevated likelihood of acquiring them. Brace yourself for the wonders that await!

Discover the Ultimate Solution to Banish Epidermis Tags!

Discover the secret to effortlessly avoiding unsightly skin tags! With our expert advice, you can significantly reduce your chances of developing these pesky blemishes. Maintain a healthy weight and say goodbye to skin tags for good! Discover the ultimate prevention tips to safeguard yourself:

- Discover the power of collaboration by teaming up with your trusted physician and a skilled dietitian. Together, you can create a personalized food plan that focuses on reducing saturated fat and calories, paving the way for a healthier lifestyle.

- Get ready to supercharge your fitness routine with our expert recommendation: engage in medium or high-intensity exercise for a minimum of 30 minutes every single day, a remarkable five times a week. Elevate your fitness game and unlock your full potential!

- Introducing the ultimate secret to maintaining flawless skin: keeping your epidermis/skin folds dry at all times. Say goodbye to friction and hello to smoothness. After every shower, make sure to gently pat your skin layer completely dry. Embrace the luxurious sensation of a perfectly dry and pampered skin. Your skin deserves nothing less than the best. Experience the ultimate freshness and comfort with our revolutionary baby powder. Gently apply our specially formulated powder to those delicate epidermis folds, such as your underarms, that are prone to trapping unwanted moisture. Embrace a feeling of dryness and confidence like never before.

Introducing our top tip for ultimate comfort: avoid wearing clothing or jewelry that causes any irritation to your precious skin layer. Embrace a world of blissful tranquility by selecting only the most gentle and soothing options for your wardrobe. Your skin deserves nothing less than pure serenity. Experience the ultimate comfort with our selection of soft, breathable materials. Opt for the luxurious feel of cotton, a fabric that surpasses the likes of nylon or spandex. Elevate your wardrobe with the perfect choice for unparalleled comfort.

Risk to Consider - Your Guide to Making Informed Decisions

Discover the secret to achieving flawless skin by understanding the factors that contribute to the formation of skin tags. One of the key factors is weight. Research shows that individuals who are overweight or obese are more prone to developing these unsightly skin tags. Take control of your skin's destiny and embark on a journey towards a healthier, more radiant complexion.

- Experience the miracle of life with our exclusive pregnancy products.

- Introducing the incredible world of type 2 diabetes!

- Discover the benefits of being in your 40s or older.

- Discover the beauty of expanding your family with

exquisite epidermis tags.

Discover the Fascinating Reasons Behind Epidermis/Skin Tags

Discover the fascinating world of skin tags, where loose collagen fibers and arteries come together, enveloped by the protective epidermis. Discover the incredible power of Collagen, a remarkable protein that naturally occurs within your body. Discover the common occurrence of skin tags in both women and men. These pesky little growths tend to appear more frequently in older individuals, as well as those who struggle with obesity or type 2 diabetes.

Experience the beauty of pregnancy with a touch of elegance. Embrace the journey of motherhood, knowing that your radiant glow may be accompanied by the occasional skin tag. These delicate adornments are simply a result of the harmonious dance of hormones within your body. Discover the mysterious allure of developing them, seemingly out of thin air. Discover the inconvenient truth about skin tags. These pesky growths have a knack for appearing in the most inconvenient places - the folds of your skin. Picture this: your skin rubbing against itself, causing irritation and discomfort. It's a common occurrence around the neck, armpits, and groin. But fear not, there's a solution. Discover the very reason why these conditions often target individuals who carry excess weight, with their abundance of folds and chafing skin.

Discover the Telltale Signs of Epidermis Tags as a Troubling Issue

Experience the peace of mind with our harmless and stress-free epidermis tags. Say goodbye to discomfort and embrace a worry-free solution. Discover the secret to boosting your self-confidence and reclaiming your flawless skin! Say goodbye to those pesky epidermis/skin tags that are holding you back. Don't let them ruin your style with constant snags on clothing or jewelry, causing painful bleeding. Take control of your appearance and invest in having them professionally removed. Don't wait any longer - it's time to put your best foot forward and feel confident in your own skin. Say goodbye to those unwanted tags and hello to a new, more confident you! Discover the secret to flawless skin with our revolutionary skin tag removal treatment. Unlike other procedures, our cosmetic surgery is designed to enhance your natural beauty. While most cosmetic surgeries are not covered by the NHS, we offer exclusive access to our state-of-the-art facilities if your skin tags are causing significant physical or mental distress. Say goodbye to unsightly skin tags and hello to a new level of confidence! Discover the fascinating world of epidermis tags, where these tiny skin growths can gracefully detach themselves when their cells undergo a natural process of twisting and perishing due to insufficient blood supply.

Experience the ultimate solution for removing unsightly epidermis tags!

Before attempting to remove an epidermis/skin tag, it is crucial to consult with your doctor for professional guidance. Discover the ultimate solution for troublesome skin tags! Say goodbye to the hassle and discomfort by scheduling a consultation with a highly skilled and dedicated privately practicing GP. Experience the relief of having your skin tag professionally removed, leaving you with smooth and flawless skin. Discover the effective methods for removing skin tags, just like the way warts are eliminated. Say goodbye to those pesky skin tags through burning or freezing techniques. Alternatively, opt for a surgical procedure with the option of a local anaesthetic for a hassle-free experience.

Experience the ultimate solution for removing unsightly skin tags! Say goodbye to freezing or burning methods that can cause irritation and temporary skin discoloration. With our innovative treatment, you can rest assured that your skin tag will be gone for good. No more worrying about it not falling off or requiring additional treatment. Trust the experts and discover the difference today!

Experience the transformative power of surgery as it effortlessly eliminates your skin imperfections. Say goodbye to skin tags with the precision and expertise of our skilled surgeons. While there may be a minimal risk of minor bleeding, rest assured that you are in safe hands. Discover the secret to effortlessly removing small skin tags with ease! Your trusted GP may suggest a simple DIY method that you can try at home. Imagine, no more hassle or inconvenience! They might recommend using dental floss or cotton to gently tie off the base of the skin tag, effectively cutting off its blood flow and causing it to naturally fall off. However, it's important to note that this method is only suitable for small skin tags with a narrow base. For larger skin tags, it's crucial to seek professional assistance to avoid any potential complications. Don't risk it! Trust the experts to handle those larger skin tags that may bleed severely. Your skin deserves the best care possible!

Chapter 2

Discover the secrets to flawless skin! Learn how to effectively remove pores and skin tags with our expert tips and techniques.

Say goodbye to unsightly blemishes and hello to a radiant complexion. Uncover the best methods for achieving smooth, clear skin that will leave you feeling confident and beautiful. Explore the world of skincare and unlock the key to a flawless appearance.

Discover the secret to effortlessly removing those pesky skin tags! While some may naturally fall off, the majority of these unsightly blemishes tend to stubbornly cling to your skin. Don't let them hold you back any longer! Introducing the remarkable world of epidermis tags! These tiny, harmless growths may not require treatment in most cases. However, if these little rascals cause you any discomfort or annoyance, fear not! You have the power to bid them farewell and have them gracefully removed.

Discover the transformative power of a skilled medical doctor who can effortlessly remove those bothersome skin tags. Experience the confidence and relief that comes from saying goodbye to those unsightly blemishes. Trust in the expertise of a professional who can delicately and effectively eliminate skin tags, leaving you with a flawless complexion. Say hello to a new you as a medical doctor expertly removes your skin tags, restoring your skin's natural beauty.

- *Introducing Cryotherapy:* The revolutionary solution to banish skin tags by freezing them with the power of liquid nitrogen.

- *Introducing our revolutionary solution for skin layer tags:* surgery. Say goodbye to those pesky tags as our skilled professionals delicately remove them using state-of-the-art scissors or a precision scalpel. Experience the freedom of flawless skin with our expert surgical techniques.

- *Introducing Electrosurgery:* The cutting-edge

method that eliminates skin tags with precision and efficiency, using the power of high-frequency electricity. Say goodbye to those unwanted skin tags and hello to flawless skin!

- *Introducing our revolutionary ligation technique:* Say goodbye to skin tags with a simple and effective procedure. By delicately tying off the tag with surgical thread, we can safely cut off its blood flow, ensuring a painless removal process. Discover the secret to effortlessly removing those pesky skin tags! While some may naturally fall off on their own, the majority of these bothersome blemishes tend to stay stubbornly attached to your precious skin. Introducing the revolutionary solution for those pesky epidermis tags! While most epidermis tags may not require treatment, we understand that some can be bothersome or even painful. That's why we offer a simple and effective way to remove them, giving you the freedom to live your life without any unnecessary distractions. Say goodbye to those pesky epidermis tags and hello to a smoother, more confident you!

- ***Introducing the pain-free solution:*** local anaesthesia. When it comes to removing those pesky epidermis tags, you won't even feel a thing. While small tags can be removed without anaesthesia, our expert medical doctors recommend using local anaesthesia for larger or multiple tags. But why stop there? We also have natural treatments that work wonders. Experience the power of tea tree oil, apple cider vinegar, and lemon juice - the ultimate trio for removing skin tags. Discover the undeniable truth: there is a lack of medical evidence to support these remedies.

Discover the daring idea of taking matters into your own hands and bidding farewell to those pesky epidermis/skin tags. Countless articles unveil the secrets of DIY techniques, such as the art of tying them off with string or indulging in a substance peel from the lime. However, it is worth noting that these methods may not be the most ideal or recommended course of action. Discover the potential risks of removing epidermis/skin tags, even in the most pristine environments. From unexpected bleeding to burns and contamination, caution is key. Leave the task to the capable hands of a medical doctor.

Discover the Secrets of Identifying Epidermis Tags

Introducing the remarkable method to effortlessly spot a skin tag - the peduncle. Unlike moles and various other skin growths, skin tags elegantly dangle from your skin's surface, thanks to this tiny stalk.

Discover the beauty of small with our collection of epidermis tags. These tiny wonders are typically smaller than 2 millimeters in size, but don't be surprised if you find some that can grow as large as many centimeters. Embrace the diversity of nature and explore the world of epidermis tags today! Experience the silky smooth touch of Epidermis tags. Discover the captivating beauty of nature's perfect imperfections. Embrace the allure of natural and circular shapes, or indulge in the charm of wrinkly and asymmetrical forms. The choice is yours to make, as you embark on a journey of aesthetic exploration. Introducing our remarkable epidermis/skin tags! These extraordinary tags are delicately threadlike, exuding an exquisite resemblance to the finest grains of grain. Experience the epitome of elegance with our exceptional skin tags.

Introducing the remarkable Epidermis/Skin Tags! These incredible tags can come in a variety of shades, from a natural flesh color to a darker tone that beautifully contrasts with the surrounding skin. This captivating effect is all thanks to the phenomenon of hyperpigmentation. Discover the beauty of Epidermis/Skin Tags today! Discover the potential consequences of a twisted epidermis/skin tag: a dramatic transformation that could lead to a striking black appearance due to insufficient blood flow.

Discover the Hidden Secrets Behind Epidermis Tags!

Discover the mysterious origins of epidermis/skin tags. Introducing our revolutionary solution: Say goodbye to discomfort caused by friction in those hard-to-reach epidermis folds. Experience the ultimate relief you deserve. Discover the fascinating composition of skin tags, where arteries and collagen intertwine within a protective layer of the epidermis.

Discover the fascinating connection between the human papillomavirus (HPV) and the development of skin tags, as revealed by a groundbreaking 2008 research. Discover the groundbreaking analysis that meticulously examined a remarkable 37 epidermis/skin tags, sourced from diverse sites across the body. Uncover the fascinating insights that await. Discover the astounding findings: HPV DNA was detected in nearly 50 percent of the skin tags that were meticulously examined.

Discover the fascinating link between insulin resistance, type 2 diabetes, prediabetes, and the emergence of skin tags. Uncover the hidden connection that could be impacting your health. Discover the secret to managing your insulin resistance and effectively absorbing blood sugar with ease. Say goodbye to the struggles of inefficient blood sugar absorption and take control of your health today. Introducing a groundbreaking 2010 study that sheds light on the fascinating correlation between multiple epidermis/skin tags and various health factors. This research has uncovered a compelling link between the presence of these skin tags and insulin resistance, elevated body mass index, and heightened triglyceride levels. Prepare to be amazed by the intriguing findings of this remarkable study!

Experience the beauty of motherhood with a touch of elegance. Embrace the natural changes that come with pregnancy, including the occasional appearance of epidermis tags. These delicate marks are a testament to the miracle of life, a result of the harmonious dance between pregnancy hormones and the graceful weight gain. Celebrate your journey and cherish every moment of this transformative experience. Discover the fascinating world of epidermis tags and their hidden meanings. In some extraordinary instances, these tiny skin growths may serve as a subtle indication of a potential hormone imbalance or an underlying endocrine issue. Unveil the secrets that lie beneath the surface.

Discover the truth about epidermis/skin tags: they are not contagious! However, there might just be a fascinating hereditary connection to these intriguing skin growths. Discover the extraordinary practice of multiple families cherishing these invaluable possessions.

Discover the Thrilling World of Risky Facts

Discover the factors that may put you at a higher risk of developing skin tags. These include being overweight, being pregnant, having a family history of skin tags, dealing with insulin resistance or type 2 diabetes, and even having HPV. Stay informed and take steps to protect your skin.

Discover the truth: Epidermis tags are harmless and do not lead to epidermis cancer. Experience the ultimate comfort with our product, where irritation becomes a thing of the past. Say goodbye to the discomfort caused by rubbing with clothing, jewellery, or other skin surfaces. Experience the ultimate precision while grooming near those delicate epidermal tags.

Discover the secret to effortlessly removing unsightly

epidermis tags without any long-term damage. Say goodbye to stress and prolonged bleeding with our innovative solution.

Discover the Optimal Time to Consult a Doctor

Discover the peace of mind you deserve by having your skin tags analyzed by a trusted physician. Don't let the uncertainty of potentially cancerous moles weigh on your mind. Remember, other common skin conditions like warts and moles can often mimic the appearance of skin tags. Take control of your health and seek professional evaluation today. Discover how your physician can expertly identify and address epidermis/skin tags. Prepare to be amazed as they effortlessly demonstrate their expertise through a meticulously designed and unmistakable examination. Discover the power of knowledge. Should any inquiries arise regarding the analysis, rest assured that a biopsy can also be performed.

Experience the ultimate in rejuvenation with our exclusive treatment. Unlock your true potential and indulge in a world of relaxation and transformation.

Discover the wonders of removing epidermis tags for a visually pleasing and aesthetically satisfying experience. Embrace the opportunity to enhance your appearance and indulge in the beauty of flawless skin. Introducing the ultimate solution for those bothersome skin tags! Say goodbye to large epidermis tags that cause discomfort when they come into contact with clothing, jewelry, or even your own pores. Experience relief from irritation as we offer a safe and effective removal process.

Experience the convenience of effortless shaving with our revolutionary skin tag removal solution. Say goodbye to the hassle of navigating around large skin tags on your face or hands. Our innovative method removes those pesky skin tags, making shaving a breeze. Embrace smooth and flawless skin with our game-changing solution.

Experience the transformative power of surgery.

Discover the array of methods at your disposal:

- *Introducing Cauterization:* Say goodbye to skin tags with the power of electrolysis! Experience the revolutionary method that burns away skin tags, leaving you with smooth and flawless skin.

- ***Introducing Cryosurgery:*** Say goodbye to unwanted skin tags with the power of freezing! Our innovative probe, filled with liquid nitrogen, gently freezes off those pesky skin tags, leaving you with smooth, flawless skin.

- ***Introducing Ligation:*** Experience the revolutionary method that interrupts blood flow to your skin layer tag.

- ***Excision:*** Experience the precision of a surgeon's scalpel as the tag is expertly sliced out.

Experience the utmost care and precision by entrusting these procedures exclusively to a highly skilled dermatologist, specialist health-care professional, or an equally qualified medical expert. Discover the ultimate solution for those bothersome epidermis/skin tags around your eyelid! Say goodbye to the hassle and discomfort with the help of a skilled ophthalmologist, a true expert in vision care. Trust the professionals to remove those unwanted tags, especially the ones near the delicate eyelid margin. Experience the relief you deserve!

Discover the safest way to remove epidermis tags in the comfort of your own home. Say goodbye to the risks of blood loss and potential infections with our expert tips. Discover the simple and effective solution for removing those pesky small tags! Say goodbye to discomfort by gently tying dental floss or a delicate cotton thread around the base of the tag. This clever technique helps cut off blood circulation to the tag, allowing it to be easily and painlessly removed.

Introducing the revolutionary world of over-the-counter solutions!

Discover the power of over-the-counter (OTC) solutions, conveniently available at your local pharmacies. These remarkable treatments freeze your skin layer tag, allowing it to gracefully fall off within just 7 to 10 days. For your peace of mind, it is recommended to seek healthcare advice before embarking on this transformative journey. Discover the incredible power of these cutting-edge medications specifically designed for effective wart removal. Say goodbye to those pesky skin tags and embrace a smoother, more flawless complexion. Rest assured, there is no evidence to suggest that removing skin tags will lead to the development of more. Experience the confidence and freedom that comes with a blemish-free skin!

Discover the effortless way to bid farewell to those bothersome skin tags! Say goodbye to the need for anesthesia when removing small epidermis tags. However, when it comes to larger or multiple tags, a skilled medical professional may opt for the use of local anesthesia. But wait, there's more! Explore the wonders of natural treatments that can help you eliminate those pesky skin tags. Unleash the power of tea tree oil, apple cider vinegar, and lemon juice to achieve flawless skin. Discover the undeniable truth: there is absolutely no medical evidence to support these remedies.

Discover the ingenious idea of tackling those pesky epidermis/skin tags on your own! Countless articles provide step-by-step DIY instructions, empowering you to bid farewell to those unwanted tags. From the daring method of tying them off with string to the revolutionary approach of applying a substance peel, the possibilities are endless. However, it is worth noting that these methods may not be the most ideal or recommended. Discover the remarkable benefits of removing epidermis/skin tags within a pristine and hygienic environment. Experience the peace of mind that comes with reducing the risk of blood loss, burns, and contamination. Why stress yourself out when you can trust the expertise of a medical doctor?

C h a p t e r 3

Discover the Ultimate Home Remedy for Effortless Skin Tag Removal!

Discover the power of consulting a trusted and knowledgeable medical practitioner before embarking on your journey to explore the following methods:

Introducing the revolutionary tag removal device!

Discover the incredible world of home remedies for skin tag removal, conveniently available for purchase online and in numerous stores. While it's true that skin tags often vanish on their own, why leave it to chance when you can opt for the swift and reliable option of medical removal?

Introducing the revolutionary unit that allows you to effortlessly acquire blood to nourish and rejuvenate your skin! Say goodbye to unsightly tags with just a simple band. The medical community refers to this incredible system as ligation, and without a reliable blood supply, those pesky cells will wither away, causing the tag to naturally disappear within a mere ten days. Experience the power of this innovative solution today!

Introducing the incredible String!

This revolutionary product is designed to meet all your string-related needs. With its exceptional durability and versatility, String is the perfect choice for any

Discover the secret to achieving ligation effortlessly with the help of oral floss or string. Don't let the challenge of doing it alone stop you - these ingenious devices or a helping hand will ensure success. With consistent use, the tag will naturally fall away after a few days of uninterrupted blood flow. Remember to tighten the string or floss daily for optimal results.

Experience the ultimate protection against infection by diligently cleansing your skin, string, and hands. Don't leave anything to chance - take the necessary precautions to keep yourself safe and healthy.

Introducing the revolutionary skin tag removal cream!

Discover the convenience of our specially curated

packages, complete with luxurious cream and a precision applicator. Elevate your skincare routine with ease and find these exclusive sets at your nearest pharmacy. Discover the secret to flawless skin with our expert-recommended skincare routine. Prepare your skin for ultimate absorption by gently cleansing with our specially formulated alcoholic wipes. Then, carefully remove the tag and unveil the true potential of our luxurious cream. Experience the difference as it effortlessly penetrates your skin, leaving it nourished and radiant. Elevate your skincare game today!

Experience the power of our cream as it gently revitalizes your skin. While it may cause a slight tingling sensation, rest assured that any tags will naturally fade away within a mere 2-3 weeks.

Introducing the revolutionary Freezing Kit!

Discover the incredible power of using a cutting-edge solution infused with the magic of liquid nitrogen to effortlessly remove those pesky skin tags. Experience the convenience of finding this remarkable product readily available at your local drugstores and pharmacies. Ensure that you carefully follow the instructions, as it may require multiple applications before a tag is successfully removed. However, rest assured that this process typically takes place within a span of ten days.

Introducing the ultimate solution for skin tag removal! Our incredible spray is designed to target those pesky skin tags without touching the surrounding epidermis. But why stop there? For an added layer of protection, we recommend applying a touch of Vaseline to the area surrounding the tag. Say goodbye to skin tags and hello to flawless skin!

Introducing the incredible Tea Tree Oil!

Introducing the miraculous Tea Tree Oil, the ultimate solution for various skin conditions, including those pesky skin tags. Say goodbye to skin troubles with this extraordinary oil. Experience the power of essential oils with our simple and effective application method. Just a few drops of our premium fundamental oil on a soft cotton ball is all it takes. Attach the cotton ball to your skin tag with a gentle bandage and let the magic happen. Leave it on for a luxurious 10 minutes, three times a day, and watch as your skin transforms. Experience the lasting power of our tags as they gracefully detach in a matter of days or even weeks.

Discover the incredible power of this treatment, but remember to handle it with care. Tea tree oil, while highly effective, can sometimes cause irritation for those with sensitive skin. Discover the secret to flawless skin with our exclusive range of essential oils. While tea tree oil is a versatile and powerful ingredient, it's important to exercise caution when applying it near the delicate eye area. For optimal results and safety, we recommend avoiding the use of tea tree oil for tags located across the eyes. Trust in our expertly curated selection of skincare products to enhance your beauty routine and achieve radiant, youthful-looking skin.

Introducing the incredible Apple Cider Vinegar!

Discover the incredible power of apple cider vinegar for removing unsightly skin tags! While research on this topic is limited, many individuals have found success by simply soaking a cotton ball in apple cider vinegar and applying it to the tag. Secure it with a bandage and leave it on for 10 minutes, repeating this process multiple times a day until the tag effortlessly falls away. Say goodbye to skin tags with the natural wonders of apple cider vinegar!

Discover the power of Iodine!

Discover the incredible power of liquid iodine in removing unsightly skin tags! Countless individuals have reported remarkable results when using this remarkable solution. Say goodbye to those pesky skin tags and embrace a smoother, more flawless complexion with the help of liquid iodine!

Introducing the ultimate skin protection solution! Safeguard your precious skin by applying a generous amount of luxurious vaseline or nourishing coconut oil to the targeted area. Experience the soothing and moisturizing benefits like never before!

Discover the secret to flawless skin with our revolutionary technique! Immerse a Q-tip in our specially formulated iodine solution and delicately apply the luxurious liquid onto your skin tag. Experience the transformative power of our innovative method today!

Protect the area with a bandage until the iodine has completely dried.

Experience the ongoing benefits of this treatment by diligently applying it twice a day until the tag effortlessly falls away.

Experience the art of precision with our cutting services.

Discover the expert-recommended method for removing unwanted skin growths: delicately trim them away with a pristine knife or scissors. However, exercise caution and avoid attempting this technique on medium or large epidermis tags, as it could potentially lead to undesirable blood loss. Discover the incredible versatility of tags, ranging from just a few millimeters to a generous 2 inches wide. These compact yet impactful tools are designed to make a lasting impression.

Discover this incredible method designed specifically for

those with delicate skin tags. With utmost care and precision, ensure that both scissors and blades are properly sterilized before and after each use. Your skin deserves nothing but the best! Discover the importance of seeking professional advice before embarking on this remarkable system. Remember, never attempt to remove epidermis or skin tags in delicate areas such as the eye or genitals without proper guidance.

Discover the perfect solution for those pesky skin tags that are causing you trouble. While home remedies can be effective for many things, they may not be the best option for skin tags located near your delicate eye area or in sensitive genital areas. It's important to find a solution that is safe and reliable.

Introducing our new and improved product:

The incredibly spacious and impressively long!

Introducing our revolutionary solution that tackles the common discomforts of pain, blood loss, and itching. Say goodbye to these pesky inconveniences with our innovative product.

Discover the power of seeking treatment in these instances. Discover the ultimate medical solutions for removing skin tags:

Introducing Cauterization: The revolutionary method that effectively removes skin tags by gently and precisely burning them away. Experience the magic as most tags gracefully disappear after just a few revitalizing treatments.

Introducing Cryotherapy: Experience the power of freezing technology as our skilled physician applies liquid nitrogen to effortlessly remove your skin tag. Say goodbye to unwanted blemishes with this innovative treatment. Experience the power of our carefully curated treatments, designed to exceed your expectations. Discover how just a few sessions can make a remarkable difference in your well-being.

Introducing our revolutionary ligation technique! Experience the incredible benefits of having the tag expertly linked off with surgical thread, resulting in reduced blood flow. Say goodbye to discomfort and hello to a smoother, more comfortable experience.

Introducing Excision: The Ultimate Solution for Tag Removal!

Discover the secret to flawless skin with our revolutionary skin tag removal treatment. Unleash your true beauty and say goodbye to those pesky skin tags. Please note that while this treatment works wonders for your confidence, it may not be covered by health insurance. Embrace your beauty today!

Discover the Perfect Time to Consult a Doctor

Discover the importance of seeking professional medical attention for large, painful, or delicate skin tags. Don't let discomfort hold you back - consult a doctor today!

Discover the importance of seeking prompt treatment for an epidermis/skin tag:

Bleeds - the ultimate solution for all your bleeding needs.

Introducing the all-new Itch-B-Gone! Say goodbye to those pesky itches that drive you crazy. With its revolutionary formula, Itch-B-Gone not only relieves itching but also transforms your skin, leaving it looking radiant and flawless. Don't let itching hold you back - experience the transformation with Itch-B-Gone today!

Chapter 4

Discover the Amazing Power of Toothpaste in Removing Skin Tags!

Introducing the revolutionary power of toothpaste! While toothpaste may not have been specifically designed to tackle those pesky epidermis tags, don't underestimate its potential. You see, toothpaste is formulated with a special ingredient - hydrogen peroxide - known for its remarkable teeth whitening properties. So, while it may not be its primary purpose, toothpaste just might surprise you with its ability to help address those skin tags. Discover the multi-functional wonders of toothpaste today! Experience the incredible benefits of hydrogen peroxide! Not only will it give you a dazzling smile, but it also has the added advantage of keeping your skin feeling fresh and dry.

Discover the secret to effortlessly removing skin tags: dry them out. Experience the power of toothpaste infused with hydrogen peroxide, as it works its magic on your skin tags. Watch in awe as these unwanted blemishes dry up and gracefully fall off, leaving you with smooth, flawless skin. Discover the essential things you need to know before reaching for the toothpaste in your medicine cabinet and applying it to your skin tags.

Discover the ultimate toothpaste experience!

Discover the crucial first step: determining the right toothpaste to effectively eliminate a skin tag. It's essential to choose the appropriate toothpaste for optimal results, as not just any toothpaste will do the trick.

Introducing the must-have toothpaste ingredient: hydrogen peroxide. Introducing our revolutionary toothpaste infused with the power of hydrogen peroxide! Experience the ultimate teeth-whitening solution with our specially formulated "whitening toothpaste"! Discover the radiant smile you've always dreamed of! Discover the power of hydrogen peroxide by simply searching for it among the list of ingredients.

Discover the remarkable difference in toothpaste quality: Experience the ultimate toothpaste innovation with our wide range of gel-based formulations. Designed to enhance your oral care routine, our toothpastes are expertly crafted for effortless application and maximum effectiveness. Discover the difference of our gel toothpastes today. Experience the ultimate in toothpaste flavor with our gel toothpaste. Indulge your taste buds with the delightful sensation of artificial flavors that will leave your mouth feeling refreshed and invigorated. Say goodbye to ordinary toothpaste and elevate your brushing routine to a whole new level of taste sensation. Experience the exquisite flavors of these artificial tastes that not only tantalize your taste buds but also make the daunting task of cleaning your teeth a bearable experience. However, it's important to note that while these flavors are irresistible to ants, they may have a slightly shorter lifespan on your skin. Discover the crucial fact: they are likely providing minimal assistance in the removal of unsightly skin tags.

Introducing the ultimate solution for tackling those stubborn skin tags - a tried and tested method that guarantees results! Say goodbye to expensive treatments and hello to a simple yet effective remedy. Our secret weapon? A classic white toothpaste, infused with the power of hydrogen peroxide. Not only does this magical formula enhance its effectiveness, but it also minimizes the risk of any unwanted side effects. And the best part? It won't break the bank! Unlike gel-based toothpaste, our recommended toothpaste is not only more affordable but also delivers superior results. Don't miss out on this game-changing solution - try it today!

Discover the Truth: Is Toothpaste Safe for Your Skin?

Experience the power of toothpaste, enriched with the incredible benefits of hydrogen peroxide. Discover a world where your skin is treated with care, as this remarkable ingredient helps to address pores, skin tags, and even combat the appearance of wrinkles. Embrace the transformative potential of toothpaste and unlock a radiant, youthful complexion. Introducing a breakthrough solution for removing skin tags without any hassle! Say goodbye to the old methods and embrace the new way. With our innovative approach, you can now apply toothpaste directly to your skin tag, ensuring a targeted and effective treatment. No more worries about unwanted side effects on your precious skin. Experience the difference today!

Discover the wisdom of opting for toothpaste, specifically the kind that contains hydrogen peroxide and is free from any artificial flavors, as we discussed earlier. Embrace the sensible choice for your dental care routine.

Discover the Ultimate Guide to Utilizing Toothpaste on Your Skin!

Discover the secret to flawless skin with our revolutionary toothpaste technique. Simply apply a small amount of toothpaste to your finger and gently massage it onto your skin tag. But beware, avoid any contact with the surrounding skin as toothpaste can be drying and may lead to unwanted wrinkles. Unlock the potential of your skin today!Never fret if a little toothpaste happens to touch your skin; simply grab a soft washcloth and gently remove any excess toothpaste with lukewarm water.

Discover the preferred method of many: applying a band-aid to your skin tag after using toothpaste. While not necessary, rest assured that this additional step will have no negative impact on your skin. Introducing our revolutionary toothpaste setup that not only stays in place but also provides a protective barrier against wiping it away.

Discover the secret to a refreshing night's sleep - the perfect bedtime routine. Join the countless individuals who have made the wise choice of incorporating toothpaste and lukewarm drinking water into their nightly rituals. Experience the soothing sensation as you cleanse your teeth before drifting off into a peaceful slumber. Discover the power of making decisions that are uniquely yours. Discover the incredible solution for those who have applied toothpaste to their skin tag. No need to worry about avoiding it before sleep anymore!

Discover the secret to a flawless skin! Find out how long it will take for your epidermis tag to gracefully fall off.

Discover the secret to removing skin tags faster than ever before! The speed at which your skin tag disappears is influenced by a variety of factors, such as the frequency of toothpaste application and the size of the skin tag itself. Unleash the power of toothpaste and say goodbye to skin tags in no time! Introducing the ultimate solution for skin tag removal! Imagine a world where those pesky skin tags simply vanish. Well, now you can make it a reality with our revolutionary method. By simply applying our specially formulated toothpaste, you can watch those skin tags disappear like magic. For optimal results, apply before bedtime and upon waking up. Say goodbye to skin tags and hello to flawless skin! Experience the ultimate sensibility by incorporating it into your daily routine, ensuring its use every few hours after indulging in a refreshing shower.

Experience a gradual yet effective transformation as the progress unfolds. With the passage of time, witness the desired outcome as it naturally fades away and effortlessly sheds. Resist the urge to hastily remove it when it begins to wither and detach. Discover the ultimate solution to eliminate skin tags once and for all! By carefully selecting the right product, you can ensure that those pesky skin tags will be completely eradicated, never to return again. Don't miss out on the opportunity to say goodbye to skin tags for good! Introducing the revolutionary solution to skin tags - say goodbye to picking and pulling! Avoid the temptation to remove them yourself and discover the safer, more effective way to deal with skin tags.

Discover the perfect solution for your skin tag with our innovative band-aid application. While it may have a slight drying effect, the effectiveness of toothpaste in removing skin tags can be a bit frustrating due to its longer removal time. Choose the best option for your needs and experience the difference. Are you tired of waiting for instant results? Well, we understand your frustration. But fear not! Our revolutionary treatment for work is here to help. Although it may require a bit of patience, the results will be well worth the wait. So why settle for quick fixes when you can experience long-lasting success? Embrace the power of patience and unlock your true potential with our exceptional treatment.

Discover the secret to flawlessly smooth skin! Say goodbye to skin tags without the worry of unsightly scars.

By opting for a prompt removal, you can enjoy the benefits of a small, permanent scar versus the alternative of a scar-free process that takes weeks. Choose the best option for your skin today!

Unleash the Power of Final Thoughts!

Introducing our revolutionary toothpaste for epidermis/skin tag removal - the ultimate choice for those seeking a more natural approach to banishing unsightly skin tags. Say goodbye to those pesky skin tags with our superb formula. Introducing our revolutionary solution that not only effectively reduces the chance of scarring, but also eliminates the need for uncertain over-the-counter products. Say goodbye to scars with our safe and reliable method. Unlock the full potential of this incredible solution by simply investing your valuable time and unwavering energy.

Discover the secret to maintaining flawless skin - avoid the perils of excessive toothpaste application. Experience the transformative power of hydrogen peroxide, a true game-changer for your skincare routine. Discover its unique ability to gently and effectively dry your skin layer, helping to combat the signs of aging and promote a youthful, radiant complexion. Embrace the future of skincare and say goodbye to wrinkles with hydrogen peroxide. Discover the essential step of ensuring that the growths are nothing but harmless epidermis tags. When it comes to your skin, uncertainty is not an option. That's why it's crucial to consult with a trusted skin specialist who can expertly address any concerns you may have. Don't take any chances with your skin's health - let a professional help you identify and treat any potential skin conditions that could be more serious.

Discover the power of nature with additional natural treatments, such as the miraculous apple cider vinegar and the potent combination of tea tree oil with coconut oil. If you're seeking alternative methods for removing skin tags, these options are worth considering. Discover the expertise of a skilled skin specialist who will guide you through a world of possibilities and address any inquiries you may have.

Chapter 5

Discover 4 Incredible DIY Methods to Eliminate Skin Tags

Introducing the ultimate solution for bothersome skin tags! If you're dealing with a non-infected tag that's nowhere near a delicate area, we've got you covered. Say goodbye to expensive treatments and hello to the convenience of treating it yourself, right in the comfort of your own home. Introducing the ultimate collection of four (4) top-notch skin tag removal methods that will revolutionize your at-home skincare routine. Brace yourself for a journey of unparalleled comfort and convenience as you explore these cutting-edge techniques. However, we must caution you that the fourth technique, while undeniably intriguing, is not recommended for home use due to its associated risks. Nevertheless, we understand the allure of curiosity, and for those daring souls who dare to venture, we present this technique for your consideration:

Experience the ultimate solution for skin layer tags - tie

them off with ease!

Introducing the revolutionary Usage Wart Remover - the ultimate solution for all your wart-related woes! Say goodbye to those pesky warts with ease and confidence. But why stop there? Elevate your wart-removal game by trying our exquisite collection of Essential Oils. These powerful oils are specially formulated to target and eliminate warts, leaving your skin smooth and flawless. And for those who prefer a more hands-on approach, we have a secret technique - scratch the tag off! Yes, you read that right. Simply scratch away the tag and watch those warts vanish before your eyes.

Discover the ultimate guide to removing skin tags with these comprehensive techniques.

Introducing Technique 1: The Revolutionary Method of Tying Your Skin Tag Off!

Introducing the revolutionary solution to effortlessly and safely eliminate those pesky skin tags right in the comfort of your own home! Say goodbye to the hassle of visiting a medical office, as tying off skin tags has become the preferred method for quick and effective removal. Until now, options for at-home removal were limited, but not anymore! Introducing an incredible solution that will revolutionize your personal hygiene routine - the Tag band Device! Say goodbye to pesky skin tags with this popular tool that is designed to prevent infection and remove them effortlessly. With our innovative skin tag removal kit, you can now easily take care of those unwanted skin tags in the comfort of your own home. Experience the convenience and effectiveness of the Tag band Device today! Introducing our revolutionary product, the ultimate solution for skin tag removal! Gone are the days of resorting to dental floss or sewing thread as a makeshift method. With our innovative product, you can now bid farewell to those pesky skin tags once and for all. Discover the downside of these procedures - they leave the spot vulnerable to illness. Introducing the remarkable sewing thread - a true force to be reckoned with. But beware, for its razor-sharp nature can leave your spot feeling more hurt and sore than ever before. Experience the undeniable discomfort that can pave the way for a heightened susceptibility to disease.

Discover the ultimate solution for eliminating those pesky skin tags with the revolutionary method of tying them off!

Proper Analysis! Always remember to consult with a trusted physician or dermatologist to confirm that the growth is indeed a harmless skin tag, and not a wart or any other potentially more serious condition.

Introducing our revolutionary spot-cleaning solution! Say goodbye to stubborn stains with our powerful detergent and water combination. Simply apply, pat dry, and experience the magic. But we don't stop there - our secret weapon is the massaging alcohol that adds an extra level of sterilization. Get ready to witness the spotless transformation!

Introducing the Stalk: Unveiling a World of Possibilities Ensure absolute clarity when determining the specific location for your disconnection.

Introducing Wrap Dental Hygiene - the ultimate solution for a healthy and radiant smile! Discover the Art of Flossing: Reach Every Corner with Ease! Experience the ultimate in secure connectivity that not only stops blood flow, but also ensures that it never compromises the integrity of your skin layer.

Introducing our revolutionary sterilization solution: Sterilize the spot daily! Say goodbye to germs and hello to a clean and safe environment. With our advanced technology, you can trust that every surface will be thoroughly sterilized, providing you with peace of mind. Don't settle for Ensure the area remains impeccably clean and shielded with a reliable bandage. Monitor the spot diligently, and apply alcohol or antibiotic cream regularly to safeguard against any potential contamination.

Discover the secret to effortlessly removing skin tags in just one week. Say goodbye to those pesky skin tags as they effortlessly fall off, leaving you with smooth and flawless skin.

Discover the Incredible Benefits of Tying Off an Epidermis Tag

Experience the convenience of getting it done in the comfort of your own home.

Introducing the ultimate skin tag removal method that will leave you amazed! With just a few simple items, you can achieve flawless results. All you need is teeth floss, rubbing alcohol, and bandages. Say goodbye to the hassle and hello to a painless experience. Don't miss out on this easy and simple solution that will have you feeling confident in no time!

Introducing the Potential Drawbacks of Tying Epidermis/Skin Tags:

Experience the possibility of irritating side effects.

Introducing our revolutionary product - the ultimate solution for your grooming needs! Discover the power of precision with our state-of-the-art device. But remember, when using this cutting-edge tool, exercise caution and avoid sensitive areas or the delicate region near your groin. Your comfort and safety are our top priorities!

Introducing our revolutionary product that guarantees to keep you safe and infection-free!

Introducing Technique 2: Harness the Power of Wart Remover!

Introducing the incredible wart removers that not only target those pesky warts, but also work wonders on unsightly skin tags! Experience the remarkable power of these removers as they effortlessly eliminate skin tags with just a single use. Introducing the ultimate solution for epidermis/skin tag removal! While not clinically proven, our cutting-edge wart removers are formulated with powerful ingredients like salicylic acid and other carefully selected elements. Discover the powerful combination of anecdotal evidence and salicylic acid, working in perfect harmony to effectively remove unsightly skin tags.

Introducing our revolutionary wart remover! Packed with the power of liquid nitrogen, the very same ingredient trusted by doctors to freeze off skin tags. With our innovative formula, you can expect remarkable results as the tag undergoes a mesmerizing transformation, changing colors before effortlessly falling off. Say goodbye to unwanted warts with our cutting-edge solution! Introducing the revolutionary wart remover that goes above and beyond - the Epidermis Tag Remover! This incredible product comes complete with a comprehensive kit, featuring a powerful cream and a convenient applicator. Say goodbye to unsightly warts and hello to flawless skin with our top-of-the-line solution.

Discover the Ultimate Solution: Skin Tag Removal with Wart Remover

Discover the Power of Proper Diagnosis: Gain the confidence you need by ensuring that the spot you are dealing with is indeed skin tags.

Introducing our revolutionary spot-cleaning solution: the perfect combination of a powerful detergent and refreshing normal water. Say goodbye to stubborn stains as you effortlessly restore the pristine condition of your belongings. Simply apply the solution, gently pat dry, and witness the magic unfold before your eyes.

Introducing the Cream Application: Experience the ultimate convenience with our easy-to-use cream. Simply follow the instructions provided and apply it with precision to achieve the desired results. Say goodbye to complicated processes and hello to a hassle-free application! Experience the luxurious benefits of our cream by applying it for a recommended duration of 20 minutes.

Experience the ultimate cleanliness with our revolutionary method: Wash and Pat Dry. Say goodbye to unwanted residue by rinsing the spot with refreshing normal water. It's time to completely eliminate the cream and embrace a spotless finish. Experience the gentle touch of our soft and absorbent pat drying technique.

Preserve the Space Impeccably Clean and Meticulously Guarded: Experience the natural healing process as a delicate scab forms after treatment. Preserve the crust with utmost care and protection until it naturally sheds in approximately three weeks.

Discover the Incredible Benefits of our Revolutionary Wart Remover for Effortlessly Removing Unsightly Skin

Tags

Discover the incredible affordability of this product. Experience the convenience and speed it offers. With just one treatment, you can bid farewell to your worries.

Discover the Hidden Drawbacks of Wart Remover for Effortlessly Banishing Skin Tags

Introducing our revolutionary task solution that guarantees results! Say goodbye to those pesky warts with our powerful formula. Experience a slight tingling sensation as our product gets to work, ensuring maximum effectiveness. While redness may occur temporarily, rest assured that it's a sign that our solution is actively targeting the problem. We understand that finding the perfect wart remover can be a challenge, but with our specially developed formula, you'll be on your way to smooth, wart-free skin in no time. Don't settle for less - choose the best!

Introducing Technique 3: Experience the Power of Essential Oils for Effortless Skin Tag Removal

Discover the incredible power of essential oils in tackling troublesome skin issues, such as skin tags. These oils are renowned for their remarkable antiseptic and antibacterial properties, making them a go-to solution for all your skin concerns. Among the many options, tea tree oil stands out as a true hero in addressing epidermis tags and other skin-related woes. Introducing the extraordinary Tea Tree Oil, sourced exclusively from the pristine Southeast Australian coastline. This remarkable essential oil is not only a powerhouse of health and wellness, but also a secret weapon for enhancing your natural beauty. Experience the incredible benefits it offers, from nourishing your skin to combating stubborn fungal infections, and even relieving bothersome coughs and congestion. Discover the wonders of Tea Tree Oil today!

Discover the wide availability of tea tree oil at numerous reputable big package stores, medication stores, and health food stores. Experience the convenience of purchasing it online. Discover the power of tea tree oil, the ultimate solution for skin tag removal. When selecting your tea tree oil, opt for a natural and 100% authentic oil that guarantees real results. Unleash the natural magic of tea tree oil as it works its wonders on your skin tags. Although it may take some time, rest assured that tea tree oil is a safe and effective method for removing those pesky skin tags. Discover the secret to achieving flawless skin with the incredible power of tea tree oil. The duration of your skin tag treatment will vary based on the frequency of application and the size of the tag itself. Say goodbye to unwanted blemishes and embrace a radiant complexion today!

Experience a noticeable difference in just 2 weeks! That's right, for many individuals, our product delivers results in record time.

Experience the power of Tea Tree Oil in eliminating unsightly epidermis tags!

Discover a multitude of solutions when harnessing the power of tea tree oil to eliminate skin tags. Unleash the potential by combining this remarkable oil with other natural powerhouses, such as apple cider vinegar.

Experience the ultimate cleanliness by meticulously cleansing your skin layer tag and the surrounding area.

Introducing the ultimate solution for your skincare routine: the cotton ball soaked in water. With its innovative design, this cotton ball is expertly crafted to deliver the perfect amount of moisture to your skin. Simply squeeze to wring out any excess water and experience the refreshing sensation as you apply it to your face. Elevate your skincare game with this must-have essential! Experience the refreshing power of tea tree oil with just three drops.

Experience the soothing relief of our revolutionary skincare solution. Simply apply our specially formulated cotton to the affected epidermis, gently massaging it over the spot for a luxurious 5 minutes. Feel the difference as our innovative product works its magic on your skin.

Experience the ultimate cleansing ritual with our gentle water wash. Delicately cleanse your skin and achieve a fresh, rejuvenated look. Simply pat dry for a flawless finish.

Discover the secret to success with this incredible technique! Experience the magic as you diligently perform this method not once, not twice, but three times a day until the tag gracefully falls off. Embrace the power of consistency and witness the amazing results unfold before your eyes.

Discover the secret to effortlessly banishing skin tags with the powerful combination of Tea Tree Oil and Apple Cider Vinegar.

Introducing the perfect blend of exquisite apple cider vinegar, refreshing lemon juice, and invigorating tea tree oil. Combine just four drops of apple cider vinegar, five drops of fresh lemon juice, and three drops of tea tree oil in a small bowl for an extraordinary experience. Experience the perfect fusion of flavors as you blend until every ingredient is harmoniously mixed together.

Experience the ultimate solution for skin tags with our revolutionary blend. Simply drop a cotton ball with this powerful formula and let it work its magic on your skin tag. Say goodbye to unwanted blemishes and hello to flawless skin.

Experience the ultimate skin tag removal with our simple yet effective method. Just gently place our soft cotton ball against the skin tag and let it work its magic for a mere 3 to 5 minutes. Say goodbye to unsightly skin tags and hello to flawless skin!

Experience the ultimate cleanliness and freshness with our revolutionary washing and drying method. Say goodbye to dirt and moisture as you indulge in the purest results. Treat your belongings to a pampering session like no other.

Experience the remarkable results by diligently following this routine twice a day for approximately ten days or until the tag effortlessly disappears.

Discover the secret to effortlessly banishing skin tags with the power of Tea Tree oil and Essential Oils!

Experience the power of nature with our invigorating tea tree oil blend. Simply combine three drops of our premium tea tree oil with a teaspoon of your favorite carrier oil, such as luxurious coconut oil or nourishing jojoba oil. Embrace the natural goodness and elevate your skincare routine to new heights. Discover the incredible power of combining it with luxurious coconut oil. Experience the ultimate skin tag removal cream, enhanced by the unique consistency of coconut oil.

Experience the soothing power of our specially crafted mixture by simply dropping a soft cotton ball into it. Then, gently massage the affected area for a few blissful moments. Feel the relief wash over you as you indulge in this luxurious self-care ritual.

Experience the ultimate cleanliness and freshness with our revolutionary washing and drying method. Say goodbye to dirt and moisture as you indulge in the purest, most immaculate results. Treat yourself to a truly exceptional experience - wash and pat dry like never before.

Discover the secret to achieving flawless skin by consistently applying this revolutionary technique until the skin tag gracefully disappears.

Discover the incredible benefits of Tea Tree Oil for effortlessly removing unsightly epidermis/skin tags.

Discover the incredible versatility of tea tree oil, a natural wonder that is not only safe for everyday use, but also suitable for pregnant women and the elderly. Rest assured, when your trusted physician gives their seal of approval, you can confidently incorporate this remarkable oil into your wellness routine. Introducing our revolutionary all-natural skin tag removal solution! Say goodbye to those pesky skin tags with our pain-free method. Experience the difference today!

Discover the Surprising Drawbacks of Tea Tree Oil for Epidermis Tag Removal

Experience the power of our unique strategy that delivers results like no other. While it may take a bit longer to work its magic, the wait is worth it. Prepare to be amazed as you delicately apply our essential oil onto the desired spot, allowing it to penetrate and work its wonders. And don't worry, we've made it easy for you to incorporate this ritual into your daily routine by providing you with the perfect amount of oil needed for multiple applications throughout the day. Embrace the journey towards your desired outcome with our exceptional product.

Introducing Technique 4: The Ultimate Solution to Remove Skin Tags!

Discover the ultimate solution to banish skin tags with this highly effective technique. However, it's important to note that attempting this method at home is not recommended. Discover the safe and effective way to remove skin tags without any risks. Don't put your health at stake by attempting to trim or scratch them off yourself. Our expert solution ensures that you avoid infections and prevent any potential bleeding. Say goodbye to the dangers and hello to a flawless skin! Discover the safest way to remove skin tags by consulting with a qualified doctor. Don't take any risks with your skin, trust the experts.

Discover the Perfect Time to Consult a Doctor for Epidermis/Skin Tag Removal

Discover the incredible power of home remedies that can work wonders in removing those pesky skin tags. However, for the utmost safety and peace of mind, it is advisable to consult a trusted doctor for professional skin tag removal. Discover the benefits of visiting a professional skin specialist for your skin tag if: • Experience the expertise of a skilled dermatologist for your new skin tag: Discover the peace of mind you deserve by having a skilled physician assess any further developments on your skin before attempting to address them at home. Discover the hidden dangers lurking in your own home. Don't let ignorance put your health at risk. Uncover the truth about potential skin cancer risks that may be silently threatening you. Take action now to protect yourself and your loved ones.

Introducing our revolutionary solution for sore or red skin tags! Discover the telltale signs that your skin tag may be harboring an unwelcome infection. Discover the secret to maintaining healthy skin by avoiding the temptation to pick at skin tags. By refraining from this habit, you can protect yourself from harmful bacteria and potential infections. Discover the telltale signs of skin tag infection: pain, swelling, redness, and a warm or hot touch. Don't hesitate - consult a doctor immediately for prompt attention.

Introducing the ultimate solution for stubborn epidermis tags that refuse to budge, even with at-home remedies: Discover the ultimate solution for those stubborn epidermis/skin tags that just won't go away at home. Discover the ultimate solution for stubborn skin tags that have withstood all your attempts at home removal. Say goodbye to those pesky skin tags and let a professional doctor take care of the job for you.

Introducing the Skin Layer Tag: A Gentle Solution for Delicate Areas! Discover how our innovative product can effectively address skin tags that may appear in sensitive areas such as near the groin and on the eyelids. Discover the secret to safely removing skin tags in delicate areas. Don't risk causing harm to your skin by attempting to remove them yourself. Trust the expertise of a qualified doctor for a safe and effective removal process.

Discover the importance of your skin layer tag: Discover the potential risks of removing a significant skin tag: excess bleeding.

Introducing our exclusive range of solutions tailored to address your specific medical ailments: Discover the safest way to bid farewell to those pesky skin tags! For individuals with blood disorders and other medical conditions, it's crucial to avoid attempting at-home methods. Why risk a potentially dangerous loss of blood? Trust the experts to provide you with the professional care you need. Discover the ultimate solution for those with a blood disorder or who are on anticoagulants - consult a doctor to effectively address and treat those bothersome skin tags.

Discover the Unveiling: A Doctor's Expertise in Removing Epidermis Tags

Are you currently facing a situation where you need assistance with epidermis/skin tag removal? If so, don't worry - we've got you covered. Our team of expert doctors is here to help you every step of the way. Say goodbye to those pesky skin tags and hello to smooth, flawless skin. Trust us, you're in good hands. Discover the essential insights on how to effortlessly eliminate skin tags during a visit to the doctor. Ease your concerns and soothe your nerves by being well-informed about what to expect.

Experience the swift and efficient removal of epidermis tags at the esteemed premises of a professional dermatologist's office: Experience the start of your appointment with a thorough examination of your skin tag by our expert dermatologist, ensuring its harmless nature. Introducing the expertise of your esteemed skin doctor, who will not only eliminate any signs of contamination but also perform a thorough cleansing of the affected area. Following this, the highly skilled dermatologist will employ one of the cutting-edge procedures to effectively remove those bothersome skin tags.

Introducing the revolutionary solution to remove skin tags: the quick and efficient method preferred by most doctors. Say goodbye to skin tags as they are expertly sliced off in the comfort of a medical office. Experience the first step of this transformative process: the meticulous cleansing of the targeted area with a powerful antiseptic solution. As the skilled physician assesses the size and location of the epidermis or skin tag, a soothing numbing solution is delicately applied to your precious skin. Introducing the skilled physician, who deftly wields a precision tool to delicately remove the unwanted tag. Introducing the incredible spot solution that will leave your clothes looking as good as new! Say goodbye to stubborn stains with our revolutionary rewashing technology. And to ensure a flawless finish, we've included a premium bandage for that extra touch of care. Experience the ultimate in spot treatment today! Experience virtually no discomfort during the procedure. Experience only a gentle pinprick sensation, while removing the tag may require the skilled hands of a physician to delicately stitch the resulting wound.

Discover the secret to effortlessly removing skin tags with the help of a skilled healthcare professional. Experience the innovative technique of freezing your skin tag using the power of liquid nitrogen. Say goodbye to unwanted skin tags and embrace a smoother, more confident you. Experience the ultimate in skin care with our revolutionary system. Watch as your skilled dermatologist expertly cleanses the targeted area, ensuring a pristine canvas for your treatment. But that's not all - we take your comfort seriously. Our exclusive numbing cream is delicately applied, ensuring a pain-free experience like no other. Experience the expertise of your dermatologist as they delicately apply a precise amount of refreshing liquid nitrogen to your skin. Experience a delightful tingling sensation as the spot gently melts away. Experience the natural process of rejuvenation as your skin layer gracefully sheds itself within a mere 10 to 14 days.

Introducing the revolutionary solution for removing skin tags: Burn Away! Say goodbye to those pesky skin tags with our cutting-edge formula. Experience the power of Burn Away and reveal smoother, clearer skin. Get ready to show off your flawless complexion! When reducing or freezing the tag off simply won't do, trust your skin doctor to expertly burn away that pesky skin tag. Experience the ultimate skin transformation as our skilled physician delicately cleanses your skin layer and its surrounding area. Using a state-of-the-art technique, a meticulously heated wire is employed to effortlessly remove the tag's stalk, leaving you with a flawless result. Discover the power of heat to protect your skin and prevent blood loss. With the help of heat, the epidermis tag will effortlessly fall off after the procedure.

Experience the hassle-free process of epidermis/skin tag removal with minimal bleeding. Introducing the revolutionary bleed-free solution for your epidermis tag removal treatment! Our skilled physicians will expertly apply a specially formulated cream to prevent any unwanted bleeding during the procedure. Say goodbye to the worry of blood loss and hello to flawless skin!

Introducing the ultimate truth about those pesky epidermis tags: while they may be annoying and unsightly, rest assured that in most cases, they are nothing more than a mere aesthetic concern, devoid of any medical implications. Discover the smart choice for removing your skin tag: consult with your insurance provider before scheduling an appointment with a physician. Discover the unfortunate truth: most insurance plans refuse to cover the cost of cosmetic epidermis/skin tag removal.

Acknowledgements

Behold the magnificent triumph of this extraordinary book, a testament to the divine intervention of God Almighty and the unwavering love and support of my cherished Family, devoted Fans, avid Readers, loyal Customers, and dear Friends. Their ceaseless encouragement has paved the way for this resounding success.

www.ingramcontent.com/pod-product-compliance
Lightning Source LLC
Chambersburg PA
CBHW031132020426
42333CB00012B/347